SOFT
AEROBICS

SOFT
AEROBICS

The New Low-Impact Workout

Nancy Burstein

A Perigee Book

Perigee Books
are published by
The Putnam Publishing Group
200 Madison Avenue
New York, NY 10016

Published simultaneously in Canada by
General Publishing Co. Limited, Toronto

Typeset by Fisher Composition, Inc.

Library of Congress Cataloging-in-Publication Data

Burstein, Nancy.
Soft aerobics.

"A Perigee book."
1. Low impact aerobic exercises.
2. Aerobic exercises—Accidents and
injuries—Prevention.   I. Title.
RA781.15.B85   1987   613.7'1   86-30533
ISBN 0-399-51360-4

Printed in the United States of America
1   2   3   4   5   6   7   8   9   10

Note

It is important that before starting any new exercise program you consult your physician. This is a must if you have any serious medical conditions or if you are taking medication. Get your doctor's consent before you begin.

While any exercise program can result in injury, low-impact soft aerobics are specifically designed to help reduce the possibility of injury from aerobic exercise.

Acknowledgments

Special thanks to Anne Edelstein, Eugene Brissie, Roger Scholl, Jim McGuire, Diane Goetz, Sanford Burstein, Susan Dresner, and U.S. Athletics.

CONTENTS

INTRODUCTION

Welcome to the newest fitness phenomenon to sweep the nation—*soft aerobics!* If you thought that jumping jacks, jogging and hopping were your only options for conditioning your cardiovascular system, then you are in for some terrific news. Aerobic dance is being revamped. No longer do you have to worry about injuries to your ankles, shins, calves, knees, hips and back. Now there is an alternative to traditional aerobics.

Soft Aerobics: The New Low-Impact Workout is your guide to the latest direction in fitness training. *Soft Aerobics* will help you understand what this new form of low-impact exercise is all about. You will learn how the dynamics of low-impact movements differ from high-impact aerobics and how to adapt soft aerobics to your individual fitness level. *Soft Aerobics* includes twelve low-impact movements that are combined into a workout of four sensational routines guaranteed to get you out of your reading chair immediately. You can even create your own soft aerobic dance combinations. You will find out how to make soft aerobics effective for losing weight as well as how soft aerobics can have an impact on preventing osteoporosis. Plus, there are lots of tips on making your low-impact program the best it can be.

If you've ever hurt yourself doing conventional aerobics, if you're concerned about the effects of high-impact work on your body, or if you're looking for a new kind of exercise experience, *Soft Aerobics: The New Low-Impact Workout* is for you. While injuries may occur in any physical activity, the movements of *Soft Aerobics* are intended to reduce the types of lower-body stress that often occur with traditional aerobics. So get ready for a gentler aerobic workout that is safe, effective and, best of all, *fun!*

1
WHAT IS SOFT AEROBICS?

As aerobic dancing became the favorite exercise regimen for over 24 million people, something interesting occurred. The activity that was supposed to keep all these exercisers fit and healthy was having an adverse side effect. A study conducted by The National Injury Prevention Foundation and San Diego State University showed that nearly 45 percent of the students of aerobic dance and 75 percent of their instructors were being sidelined with injuries. All of the bouncing, hopping and jumping movements were creating continued stress on the lower body that was beyond what the musculoskeletal system is designed to absorb.

In response to this situation, the fitness industry began to take a closer look at aerobics classes. What would happen if all those high-powered jumps and hops were replaced with softer, gentler movements? Would it still be possible to obtain a cardiovascular benefit? Could aerobics classes be as dynamic and fun with lower-impact routines?

There is lots of good news! First, it is possible to achieve aerobic conditioning without jumping up and down, and second, a class that comprises gentler moves can be just as enjoyable as a traditional aerobics class. In fact, many of the familiar movements of high-impact routines can be adapted for soft aerobics.

So what exactly is soft aerobics and how does it differ from high-impact aerobics? With soft or low-impact aerobics, one foot always remains in contact with the floor. Since motions with elevation are eliminated, there is less compression to the body because the amount of vertical force on the feet (as they touch the floor) is decreased. To help elevate the heart rate, there's more emphasis on bending motions that use the large leg muscles (the thighs and buttocks) and on actions of the upper body to make the cardiovascular system work harder.

By contrast, high-impact movements using jumps, hops, skips and jogging create an increased vertical force on the body. The high-impact routines are effective in raising a participant's heart rate for aerobic benefits—but at a cost. The repetition of the ballistic motions can create an "overuse" syndrome that means injuries to the muscles, joints and bones.

To distinguish between high-impact and soft aerobics, think about the differences between two other forms of aerobic exercise—jogging and racewalking. Jogging is high-impact exercise: in the moment between strides, both feet are off the ground at the same time. The jogger achieves a moderate amount of elevation, and, while the arms are moving, the primary action occurs in the legs. Each time the foot hits the ground, the vertical force considerably exceeds the weight of the body.

Racewalking, however, is a low-impact activity during which one foot always stays in contact with the ground. There is no elevation. Racewalkers place a greater emphasis on motions of the hips and continual pumping of the arms to propel the body.

Soft aerobics can be described as using the muscles rather than pounding the joints repetitively with jumping actions. Each lower-body movement is cushioned to reduce stress on the legs, hips and back. Low-impact routines accentuate the use of the upper body—motions of the arms such as biceps curls, arm presses in all directions and triceps work—to make the heart work harder and help the participant achieve a cardiovascular training effect from the workout.

WHY SOFT AEROBICS?

Are you or have you ever been an "exercise drop-out"? For the uninitiated, exercise drop-outs are those individuals who begin an exercise program and within a short time discard the activity to return to the familiar, albeit unhealthy, security of sedentary living. The drop-out syndrome occurs for various reasons, but these are common refrains:

"I hurt myself, and obviously this body is not meant for exercise."

"I couldn't keep up with the rest of the class and felt like a failure."

"I never knew I would be so sore! It's not worth the discomfort."

It's pointless to continue an activity that injures you, makes you feel inadequate or pushes you too quickly to do too much. That's why it's critical to select an activity that reduces your risk of injury, gives you a sense of accomplishment and offers options for increasing the intensity gradually.

WHO CAN BENEFIT FROM SOFT AEROBICS?

Soft aerobics can be done safely and effectively by any healthy individual. The beauty of the program is its ability to offer a fitness challenge to the newcomer to exercise as well as to the more experienced participant. It's an activity appropriate to all age groups and both sexes.

Beginning Exercisers

The novice exerciser who has found traditional aerobics classes too rigorous to sustain will discover that low-impact routines are doable. The intensity of this program can be adapted to suit the individual, and the beginner can start by first executing the leg movements and then gradually including motions of the upper body. Many of the low-impact routines are based on uncomplicated foot and arm patterns that are easily learned. Because soft aerobics emphasizes a variety of arm gestures, the participant will strengthen the upper body in addition to the cardiovascular system.

Injured Exercisers

For exercisers who have suffered injuries, soft aerobics offers a road back to a regular regimen of activity that can be accomplished without pain or stress to the lower limbs. It is ideal for people with orthopedic problems who may have dismissed the possibility of ever again participating in an aerobics class.

The Overweight

Aerobic exercise is an important factor in weight-control programs. However, overweight people generally have difficulty locating aerobics classes suitable for their needs. The high intensity of traditional classes creates too much stress on the body. Soft aerobics, with its gentler, cushioning movements, can be a successful choice for the overweight. Soft aerobics are also recommended for large-breasted women who find traditional aerobic exercise uncomfortable.

Pregnant Women

Conventional aerobics have been discouraged for pregnant women, and rightly so. Bouncing, jerky motions are contraindicated during pregnancy. While the expectant mother must check with her physician before engaging in any exercise program, most doctors maintain that a program of moderate activity is safe. Pregnant women often find they can continue their regular aerobics program if they switch to low-impact routines.

Older Exercisers

Middle-aged or elderly individuals who don't get regular exercise may think it is too late to start now. The truth is, it's never too late to begin exercising. But it's prudent to consider what kind of exercise is most appropriate and what activity can be initiated safely in later years. With the reduced impact of soft aerobics, exercise can be gentle and satisfying for the older person.

By now, the experienced exerciser may be thinking, "How can I achieve fitness benefits from this gentler form of aerobics?" The unique quality of soft aerobics is its adaptability to all fitness levels. The more advanced individual can use light weights (one to two pounds) for the upper body to add resistance and create greater intensity.

2
CARDIO-VASCULAR CONDITIONING WITH LOW-IMPACT AEROBICS

Working the heart. If you have time for only one fitness activity, physicians and exercise specialists alike recommend that you make it aerobic. Cardiovascular health is a priority, but not if it is achieved at the expense of an injury. What good is the most conditioned cardiovascular system if stress to your joints, muscles or bones eventually prevents you from continuing the activity? Soft aerobics can effectively condition the heart and lungs without compromising the body's musculoskeletal system.

Aerobic is defined as "living, active or occurring only in the presence of oxygen." As it relates to exercise, it is energy production in the body (actually the cells) that requires oxygen. Aerobic exercise is any exercise that uses large muscle groups of the body (e.g., thighs, buttocks, back), usually in a rhythmic manner, that is performed for a prolonged period of time (at least fifteen minutes). It conditions your heart and lungs by increasing the oxygen available to your body and enabling your heart to use oxygen more efficiently.

THE BENEFITS OF AEROBIC CONDITIONING

Aerobic exercise offers a wealth of benefits that affect your health and well-being. Here are some of the ways soft aerobics can keep you fit in the short term and the long term:

- Aerobic exercise is a major factor in fighting cardiovascular disease.
  A regular program of soft aerobics will help lower blood pressure and make the heart work more efficiently. Over a period of time, the resting heart rate and the exercise heart rate will also decrease. In addition, the level in the blood of HDL (high density lipoprotein) cholesterol, the good cholesterol, generally rises.
- Aerobic exercise burns calories.
  Soft aerobics can be a key factor in weight control. A low-impact/moderate-intensity workout will more effectively burn body fat and have a positive effect on body composition (the ratio of fat tissue in the body to lean body mass, which is

the muscles, bones, organs and connective tissues.)

- Aerobic exercise is a successful tool in counteracting stress.

  Soft aerobics provides a physical release for the tension the body's muscles produce during a pressured, stressful day. During aerobic activity, the body releases a chemical called beta-endorphin, a mood elevator more powerful than morphine, that alleviates depression and creates a sense of euphoria.

In addition to the above benefits, soft aerobics can also reduce the rate of bone mineral loss that may lead to osteoporosis, reduce overuse syndrome (injuries that result from repetitive movements creating excessive stress on the body), and even help control diabetes.

AEROBIC EXERCISE GUIDELINES

Before you embark on a low-impact program, here are some basic exercise principles and guidelines for safe aerobics. The greater your understanding of what constitutes fitness, the better equipped you are to gain maximum benefits from your soft aerobics workout. The concepts of *overload*, *frequency*, *intensity* and *duration* are fundamental in creating appropriate training levels for all exercisers.

Overload simply means that to increase your cardiovascular endurance, you must push your body beyond its normal capacity or regular workload. For example, if you can comfortably perform ten minutes of low-impact aerobics, to improve your stamina you must increase the amount of time you exercise. You could accomplish this by adding one or two minutes to your routine every couple of weeks. If you are an experienced aerobic exerciser, adding light weights for the upper body is another way to increase the workload. Progression is a necessary factor that prevents overexertion while gradually conditioning the body.

Overload and progression are related to three specific exercise guidelines for soft aerobics:

1. Frequency

To achieve an aerobic conditioning effect, or training effect, you must exercise at least three times a week. This training effect is the response of the body to the overload of training. It results in gains such as a lowered resting heart rate and improved oxygen consumption.

2. Intensity

For the training effect to occur, your heart rate must reach a level of intensity known as your target zone.

3. Duration

The activity session must last for at least fifteen minutes to elicit a training response.

THE TARGET HEART-RATE ZONE

While most exercisers know how many days a week they exercise and for how long, intensity is often overlooked. The degree of intensity is an indication of how hard you are working and should be measured at regular intervals during the activity session. You must work hard enough to achieve a training effect without going above your appropriate training level. Your pulse can tell you whether you are exercising too hard, not hard enough, or at the right level to improve cardiovascular fitness.

Guidelines for target heart-rate zones vary according to different national health organizations. The American Heart Association calls for a target zone of 60 percent to 75 percent of the maximum heart rate, while the American College of Sports Medicine states that the heart rate may go up to 90 percent of the maximum. For most people it is generally best not to exceed 85 percent. If you are just beginning an aerobic program, you should progress gradually, beginning at 60 percent of your maximum. After six months or more of regular exercise, you can exercise at up to 85 percent of your maximum heart rate if you wish. However, you do not have to exercise that hard to stay in good condition.

An intensity of 60 to 75 percent still produces a training effect but diminishes the chance of orthopedic problems and cardiac dysrhythmias (irregular heartbeats). While high-impact movements involving jumps and hops can elevate the heart rate to a higher range, they create added stress to the joints.

MONITORING YOUR HEART RATE

You can calculate your target heart-rate zone with the following formula based on age:

220 minus your age	= maximum heart rate
maximum heart rate × .60	= low end of target zone
maximum heart rate × .75	= high end of target zone

For example, the calculation for a 35-year-old is:

$$220 - 35 \quad = 185 \text{ (beats per minute)}$$
$$185 \times .60 \quad = 111$$
$$185 \times .75 \quad = 139$$

The target zone for a 35-year-old man or woman is 111 to 139 beats per minute.

Calculate your target zone with the formula:

220 − _____ (your age)   = _____ (beats per minute)

_____ (beats/min) × .60   = _____ (low end)

_____ (beats/min) × .75   = _____ (high end)

The following table will give you the target zone closest to your age.

TARGET HEART-RATE ZONE

Use the target zone for the category closest to your age.

Age	Target Zone	
	60–75%	*75–85%*
20	120–150	150–170
25	117–146	146–166
30	114–142	142–162
35	111–138	138–157
40	108–135	135–153
45	105–131	131–149
50	102–127	127–145
55	99–123	123–140
60	96–120	120–136
65	93–116	116–132

While you are doing soft aerobics, you can check your pulse to see how many times per minute your heart is beating. Take your pulse by placing the tips of your first two fingers on the inside of your wrist at the radial artery or on one of the carotid arteries located on either side of the neck under the jaw. (If you choose to take a pulse at the carotid artery, it is important that the fingertip pressure be gentle. Excessive pressure can cause the heart rate to slow down and, in extreme cases, may cause unconsciousness.) Count the beats for ten seconds and multiply by six. This gives you the number of heartbeats per minute. If you take your pulse for longer than ten seconds, your heart rate will begin to slow down and will not give you an accurate indication of whether you were in your target zone.

As you monitor your heart rate during the low-impact routines, be sure to keep the body moving rather than stopping abruptly. When movement ceases blood can pool in the working limbs and possibly cause lightheadedness. Walking in place or around the room while taking a pulse is the easiest way to keep the body moving.

PERCEIVED EXERTION

Taking a pulse rate to monitor how hard you are working during the low-impact routines is an excellent method for measuring intensity. For some participants, particularly those who have difficulty finding their pulse and persons who take medication for high blood pressure, the technique of estimating perceived exertion provides a better measuring tool.

With the perceived-exertion method, you estimate how much work you are doing by sensitizing yourself to the reactions of your body. This is also referred to as "listening to the body."

Using the following scale, ask yourself, "How hard am I working?"

Perceived Exertion Scale

1
  very, very light
2

3 very light

4
  fairly light
5

6 somewhat hard

7 hard

8
  very hard
9

10 very, very hard

A perceived exertion that ranges from 6 to 8 is generally an indication that you are achieving a cardiovascular training effect. While it may seem that perceived exertion is too subjective a method to measure intensity accurately, studies have shown that it correlates closely with target heart-rate zones when pulses are taken.

Along with perceived exertion, try the talk test to be sure that you don't go above your target zone. If you can carry on a conversation without panting or gasping for air during the soft aerobics routines, you are probably working within your appropriate range.

3

USING THE UPPER BODY AND LIGHT WEIGHTS IN SOFT AEROBICS

Most people get adequate lower-body exercise in the course of their normal routines (walking, climbing stairs, etc.). They rarely get upper-body exercise unless they seek it out. The use of the upper body is an identifying characteristic of soft aerobics. Movements of the arms can elevate the cardiovascular load considerably without added stress to the legs. For many participants, simply keeping the arms active with various gestures (while the feet are executing low-impact movements) will elevate the heart rate to a target zone. In addition to the cardiovascular benefits, all of the arm, chest, shoulder and back movements contribute to stronger muscles and a toned appearance. Well-conditioned exercisers, however, may need to include light weights, hand-held or wrist models, in their workouts to make the upper body work harder and increase the cardiovascular load.

With any arm or upper-body motions, whether or not you use weights, your movements must be done carefully to avoid injury. If they are done too quickly, you will create a force and momentum that can take a limb beyond its normal range of motion in the joint. Repeated actions of this sort may cause a host of ligament, tendon and joint problems. To control your movements, think of moving your arms as if they were under water.

If you are new to a soft aerobics program, follow the workout for several weeks in order to master the arm movements before deciding whether or not to add weights. *Note:* People with hypertension, joint or orthopedic problems should consult their physician before doing any type of work with weights.

While working with weights will help to increase muscular endurance, it will not produce large, bulky muscles. You develop bulk by lifting heavy weights for several repetitions, as in weight training or body building. In soft aerobics, the light weights will simply give your muscles more definition and your body lots more stamina.

WHAT YOU NEED TO KNOW ABOUT LIGHT WEIGHTS

1. Weights for low-impact aerobics are available as small dumbbells, slip-on wrist models or wraparound styles that may also be held in the hands.

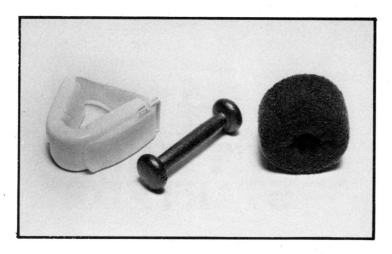

2. Weights of one or two pounds should be used for soft aerobics. Most people can achieve a training effect with one-pound weights.

3. If you want to use heavier weights, start with one pound and add weight in one-half to one pound increments. Don't increase the weight until you can perform the low-impact routines without fatigue to your muscles.

4. If you are using hand-held weights, hold them securely but don't grip them tightly. Tightly gripped hands and fingers can restrict blood flow.

5. Never use light weights on the ankles for low-impact aerobics. The added weight can over-stress the muscles and joints, resulting in ankle, calf or knee injuries.

6. Do not use weights during the warm-up for soft aerobics—or any type of exercise, for that matter. During a warm-up, you want to prepare the muscles and joints for movement without the added resistance of extra weight.

4
GETTING STARTED

There's nothing like the anticipation of beginning a new exercise program. Getting geared up for its challenges and pleasures makes many of us want to get going pronto! Getting Started will help you make Soft Aerobics the best it can be, with suggestions and tips for a successful and satisfying workout.

FLOORS AND FOOTWEAR

What you dance on and what you dance in are as important as what dance steps you do. Injuries caused by traditional aerobics are not only the result of high-impact movements. Exercising on inappropriate surfaces and using improper footwear have been cited as possible causes for lower-body problems.

Floors: Nonresilient surfaces such as concrete, linoleum, or concrete covered with carpet should never be used for *high*-impact aerobics. These floors provide no "give" and will not cushion the vertical impact created by a jump or hop. Good surfaces for high-impact dancing are padded floors (a layer of foam between the subflooring and covered by carpet, vinyl or wood) or spring floors (coiled springs topped with wood or carpet).

Because the movements of soft aerobics are designed to decrease impact stress, the vertical absorption characteristics of a surface are not as crucial. There is another consideration, however. Many low-impact movements are lateral or side to side, creating significant surface friction. A thick, padded carpet might dissipate vertical stress, but its traction properties would severely inhibit a gliding step or pivoting motion. Smooth hardwood floors are the best surfaces for soft aerobics because they provide stable support and reduce foot drag or friction.

Footwear: The first question often asked about shoes is, "Are they necessary for soft aerobics?" The answer is Yes. Soft aerobics is low-impact exercise, and, although there is less impact than with traditional aerobics, some amount of vertical force still exists. The cushioning provided by appropriate shoes offers additional protection for your muscles and joints.

Barely five years ago there were no shoes specifically designed for aerobics. Now the choices are numerous, and trying to select one pair from a display of dozens can be daunting. While the choice of footwear is an individual one, here are some criteria suggested by the International Dance-Exercise Association for choosing shoes best suited for a low-impact program.

1. Fit and comfort are the cornerstones of the shoe

that's best for you. Try on various models, and, if you use orthotics, be sure to bring them along.

2. Soft aerobics performed on a carpeted surface requires a smoother sole that reduces traction and allows for more foot glide. A shoe with more tread can be used on a smooth surface such as vinyl or wood.

3. The shock-absorption qualities of a shoe provide impact protection. Mid-soles constructed with a pocket of air to cushion the feet or those designed with a lightweight man-made material called ethylene vinyl acetate (EVA) will effectively protect against impact. Too much cushioning can affect your balance during workouts, however, and should be avoided.

4. Look for shoes that will give you lateral support and stability. A straight last (the outsole upon which the shoe is built) provides a more secure base than a narrow, curved type. Side straps or reinforcements provide lateral and medial support for the outer and inner sides of the feet. A rigid heel counter at the back of the shoe that holds the foot in place aids stability.

5. To obtain maximum wear from your shoes, wear them only in aerobics classes.

6. No shoes will last forever, but those used only for soft aerobics will have a longer life than ones used for high-impact work. Examine your shoes after six months of wear to evaluate whether they need to be replaced. Although the tops of the shoes may appear to be in good condition, check the amount of compression in the cushioning layer. It can be helpful to measure this when the shoes are new for comparison purposes.

WHAT TO WEAR

If the variety of shoe styles seems awesome, the possibilities for bodywear are staggering. Although you can't open a fashion magazine without seeing the latest in exercise gear, new workout clothes are not a prerequisite for exercising. They may help motivate a reluctant exerciser or be a reward for achieving fitness goals, but it's not necessary to spend lots of money in order to exercise.

When deciding what to wear for soft aerobics, the key word is comfort. Clothing that allows ease of motion and enables you to see how your body is moving is the best choice. Leotards and tights, bodysuits, shorts and t-shirts, sweat clothes or loose pants and a top can all work effectively. Avoid bulky clothes that prevent you from seeing body alignment.

You may want to consider layers of clothing that can be removed as your muscles become warm and pliant. An extra t-shirt or sweater can come off once you're partway into the workout. Some people find that until their core body temperature rises, a pair of sweatpants over tights offers added warmth to the legs and hips. The Achilles tendons and calf muscles can be kept warm throughout the workout with high socks or leg warmers. You are less likely to strain your muscles when they are kept warm.

Most importantly, choose something that makes you feel good about yourself and ready to have some fun exercising.

MUSIC

Music to accompany soft aerobics is an important factor in a workout. It not only enhances the routines, but it also can be the stimulus to get you off the sofa and into the exercise spirit. The music you choose must have two qualities: it must make you want to move, and it must have an appropriate tempo that enables you to execute the movements correctly.

Although popular music is generally used to accompany aerobics routines, there are many more options available. Consider trying jazz, big band, country, show tunes or even classical music for a change. A broad range of selections can give pizzazz to your fitness program.

Throughout low-impact aerobics, the quality of resistance is emphasized. Movements must be controlled to avoid momentum taking over from muscle action. Resistance and control, along with proper body alignment, can best be achieved with a music speed a bit slower than that used in traditional aerobics.

Music speed is determined by the number of beats per minute. The Aerobics and Fitness Association of America recommends that low-impact routines use music with 125 to 145 beats per minute. If light weights are used, the speed should be slightly slower, 120 to 140 beats per minute. You can easily calculate whether your favorite tunes are suitable for soft aerobics by counting the beats of music in the first ten seconds of the song and multiplying that figure by six. If you select music with a faster speed, be sure to make all movements smaller to avoid jerking the body.

MAKING YOUR EXERCISE PROGRAM A SUCCESS

Exercising at home is the ultimate in convenience. You don't have to adjust your schedule to class times at health clubs or exercise salons, and travel time is eliminated. It's the best bargain around, too, since there are no membership costs, yearly dues or class fees. However, unless you make exercise a priority in your schedule, it's easy to keep saying "I'll start tomorrow." With just a little forethought, you can guarantee that exercise will become a part of your lifestyle.

First, if you have not been exercising regularly, be patient and exercise moderately. Fitness gains are not achieved overnight. The muscles, joints, bones, ligaments and tendons need to be eased into activity gradually and carefully. There's no need to experience extreme stiffness and soreness the day after exercise. It's better to do a little less initially than to overdo and become discouraged.

Set aside a regular time in your day for exercise. Sometimes it's helpful to write the exercise session in your calendar as though it were an appointment. Once exercise is given the same priority as a business meeting, doctor's appointment or social engagement, there's less chance that it will be canceled or postponed.

If you're an early-morning riser, getting out of bed into workout gear for some "rise and shine" soft aerobics is a terrific way to start the day. A noontime or afterwork exercise session provides a boost that will increase your energy level for the rest of the day. The only time not recommended for aerobic exercise is the late evening, because the invigorating activity may make falling asleep difficult.

The following Body Basics checklist offers additional recommendations for a safe, beneficial workout.

1. Avoid eating one and one-half to two hours before exercising. Besides making you feel uncomfortable, too much food in the digestive tract can cause cramping during exercise.
2. Drink water before, during and after your workout to prevent dehydration caused by the loss of fluids through sweating. Salt tablets, however, are unnecessary and unhealthy.
3. During exercise, there is a tendency to hold your breath unconsciously. Be sure to breathe regularly in order to bring a continuous flow of oxygen to the muscles through steady inhalations and exhalations.
4. If at any time during the workout you feel pain, stop immediately. Pain is a signal that something is wrong and that the movement should be discontinued. If the pain persists, check with your physician.
5. Throughout soft aerobics, your abdominal muscles should be pulled in and lifted to give support to your torso and lower back. Strong abdominals contribute to good posture and help prevent back problems.
6. As you straighten your legs during various movements, always keep your knees relaxed. Never "jam" or "lock" your knees; this action causes hyperextension that strains the ligaments and tendons of the joint. This principle also applies to the elbows.

7. Your shoulders should be relaxed throughout a workout. Hunched or lifted shoulders create muscle tension that inhibits the proper execution of upper-body movements. Watch yourself in a full-length mirror occasionally to check your form.

DOING SOFT AEROBICS AT A HEALTH CLUB OR EXERCISE STUDIO

Outside group classes can be a nice supplement to exercising alone. Group classes offer the opportunity for instruction on body alignment and the chance to try out different routines. The camaraderie of a class can also be fun and provide motivation to exercise. However, the rapid proliferation of health clubs and exercise salons raises the question of instructor competency. In some cases, the instructor leading a class may not have the proper qualifications or training to be teaching exercise.

Before joining a group class, inquire about the background of the instructor. A teacher with a degree in exercise physiology, dance education or physical education, or one who has been certified to teach dance exercise, has demonstrated an understanding of movement principles and fitness training. Instructors with degrees or certifications have generally studied anatomy and kinesiology, exercise physiology, injury prevention, correct exercise execution and teaching techniques. The American College of Sports Medicine, The International Dance-Exercise Association and The Aerobics and Fitness Association of America are three certifying organizations recognized by professionals in the field.

5
WARMING UP FOR THE LOW-IMPACT WORKOUT

Once you're ready to start exercising, the temptation may be strong to get right into the soft aerobics and skip all of the pre-aerobic warm-ups. Temper that temptation! The warm-up is an absolute necessity, giving your body time to prepare for the more vigorous upcoming activity. If you've ignored the warm-up phase of exercising in the past, now's the time for a new resolution.

Warm-up exercises are one of the key factors in minimizing the possibility of injury. By increasing circulation and generating a greater blood flow to the body's extremities, warm-ups raise the body's core temperature slightly and literally "warm" the muscles. Warm muscles are pliant, and they can move more freely than "cold" muscles, which resist movement. Warm-up exercises also improve the flexibility of the ligaments and tendons, and increase joint mobility.

You can warm up sufficiently in five to ten minutes. On the days when you are feeling particularly stiff, take a little more time. Listen to your body and give extra attention to those muscle groups that are tight or tense.

The following warm-up exercises will help prepare your body for the low-impact workout.

THE TWO-MINUTE WALK AROUND

1. One of the most effective ways to increase circulation and body temperature is to move the entire body in a gentle, nonstressful manner. A brisk walk around the room or an easy march in place with the arms pumping will make the muscles more responsive to the next sequence of exercises for specific muscle groups.
2. Play your favorite record as you do the walk around, to set the spirit for the rest of your routine.

NECK STRETCH WITH HEAD ROLL

1. Tilt head to the right, bringing right ear close to shoulder.
2. Drop the chin to the chest and roll the head to the left making a half-circle.
3. Return the head to an upright position.
4. Reverse by tilting head to the left and continue with head roll to the right.

   Repeat 4 times.

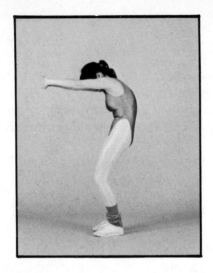

SPINE STRETCH

1. Standing with feet about hip-width apart, bend knees and make a "C" shape with the torso. The hands are clasped with the arms pressing straight forward to accentuate the stretch. The neck is relaxed and the chin is dropped toward the chest.
2. Hold the stretch for ten seconds, release and repeat.

SHOULDER ROTATIONS

1. With arms down at sides, push both shoulders forward.
2. Lift the shoulders up toward the ears.
3. Press the shoulders back.
4. Relax the shoulders down.
5. Reverse by starting backward.

   Repeat 4 times.

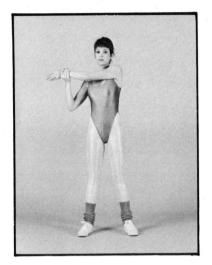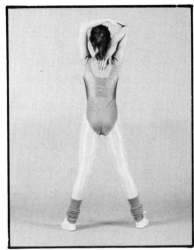

DELTOID (SHOULDER) STRETCH

1. Holding the left wrist with the right hand, pull the left arm across the chest.
2. Hold for 15 seconds.
3. Change arms and repeat stretch.

TRICEPS (BACK OF THE UPPER ARM) STRETCH

1. Both arms are bent above the head. Place the right hand on the upper back between the shoulder blades. With the left hand, gently pull the right elbow toward the head to stretch the right triceps muscle.
2. Hold the stretch for 15 seconds.
3. Change arms and repeat.

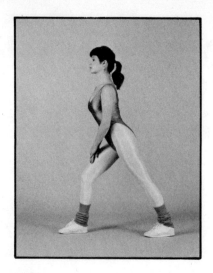

CALF STRETCH

1. Standing in a lunge position, bend the right knee and extend the left leg. Both feet are pointed forward and the left heel is raised slightly.
2. Gently press the left heel toward the floor. Hold the stretch for 20 seconds.
3. Repeat with the right leg extended back.

TORSO STRETCH

1. Stretch both arms above the head and imagine you are grabbing onto the rung of a ladder with the right hand.
2. Stretch the left hand higher than the right.
3. Continue the "climbing" motion and alternate the arms.

   Repeat 8 times.

6
THE BASIC MOVEMENTS

The Low-Impact Workout consists of twelve basic movements that are combined to create four different routines. Once you have mastered the core movements, you can follow the routines presented here or create your own arrangements. The key is to enjoy yourself and to make your workout energetic, spirited and *fun*. So, let's go!

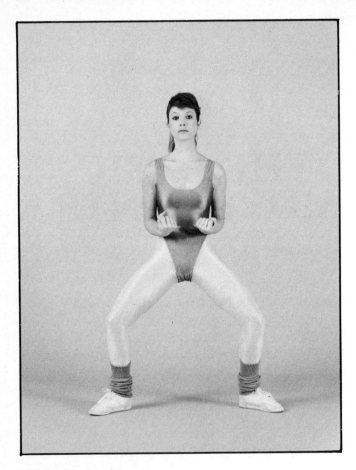

PENDULUM PUSH

1. Legs are shoulder-width apart, with the knees
   bent and the feet turned out slightly. (The
   abdominal muscles are pulled in and the lower
   back is lengthened. No arching, please!) Arms are
   bent, elbows back and forearms at waist.

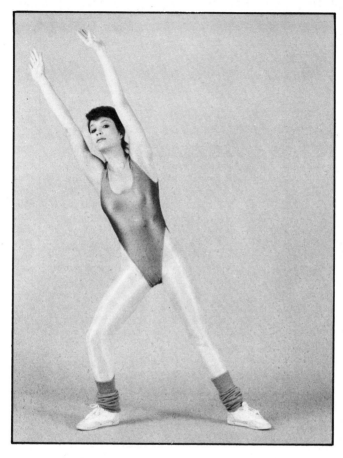

2. Shift your weight to the right as you straighten
   your left leg. At the same time, push your arms in
   a controlled motion to the upper right diagonal.

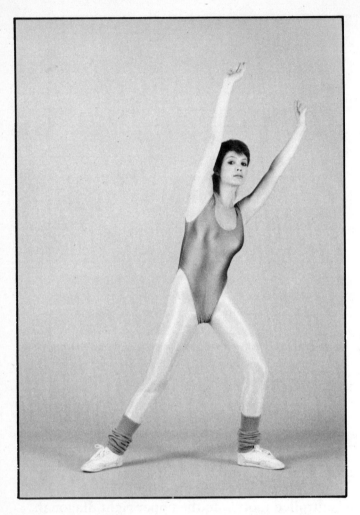

3. In one fluid movement, return to the starting
   position and then shift to the left.

Each push from one side to the other is one repetition.
Do 24 pushes.

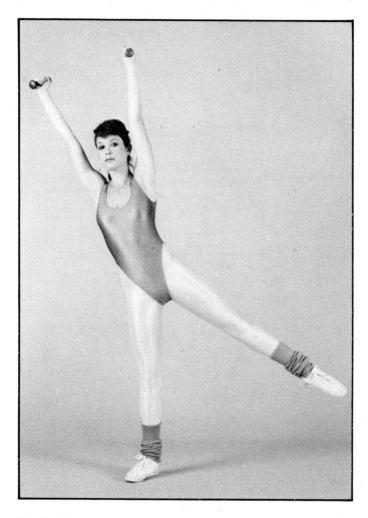

Variation

As the body shifts to the right side, straighten both legs and lift the left foot off the floor. Repeat to the opposite side.

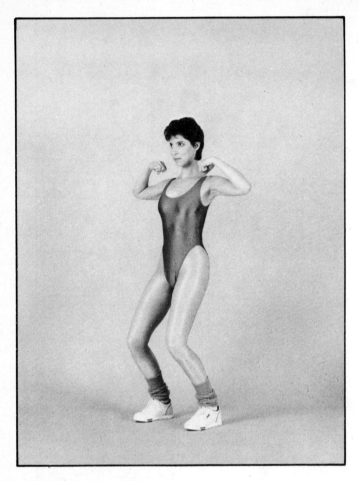

CHORUS LINE SPECIAL

1. Stand with feet hip-width apart and knees bent. Lift arms to shoulder level and bend elbows, bringing fists to shoulders.

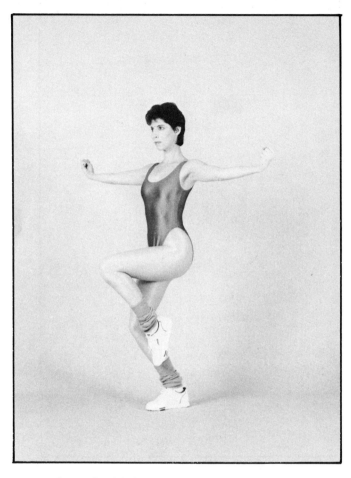

2. Angling the body slightly to the right, lift the left knee and touch left foot to the right calf as you straighten the arms.
3. Return to the starting position.
4. Repeat to the other side by bending right knee and touching right foot to the left calf.

Alternating sides, do 16 times.

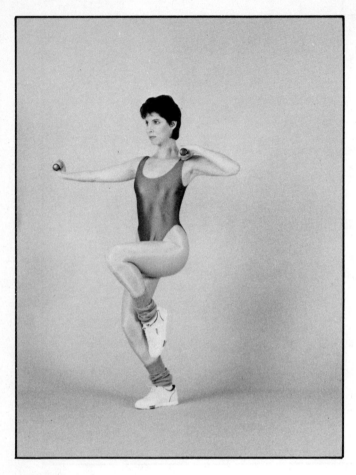

Variation

As the left knee lifts, straighten only the right arm. The left arm will straighten when the right knee lifts.

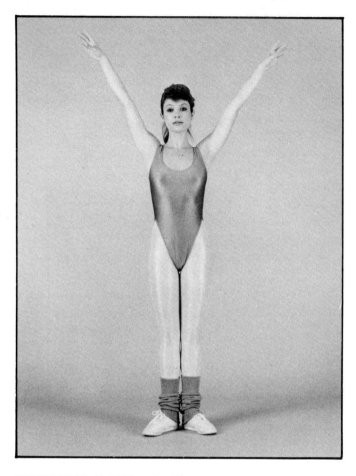

THE PULL-DOWN KNEE LIFT

1. Standing with the legs together and straight, turn out the feet slightly. Arms are extended straight above the head.

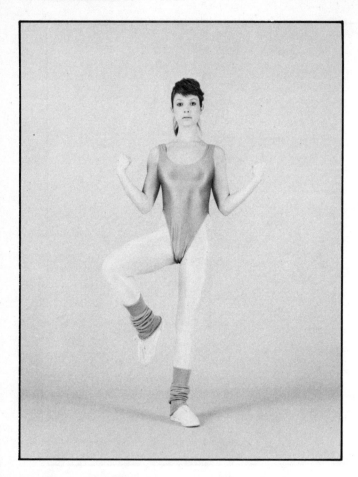

2. Lift the right knee to the right side (keep the back straight and tummy tucked in) as you pull the arms down and bend the elbows. The knee does not have to touch the elbow.
3. Return to the starting position.
4. Repeat to the left side by lifting the left knee as the arms pull down and elbows bend.

Do 16 repetitions.

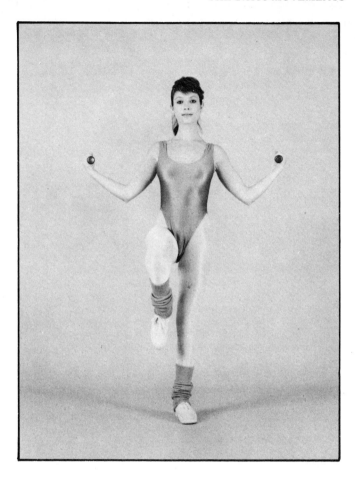

Variation

Place the feet in a parallel position (toes pointing straight forward) hip-width apart. As the arms pull down, lift the right knee in front of the body. Repeat with the left knee.

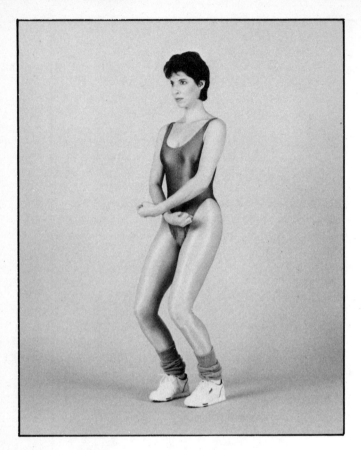

HALF JACKS

1. Stand with the legs together, knees slightly bent
   and arms crossed in front of body with hands
   closed into fists.
2. Stretch the right leg to the side and touch the
   right heel to the floor (the toes point to the
   ceiling) as you lift arms up to shoulder level.
3. Press the arms down to the sides as the legs
   return to the starting position.

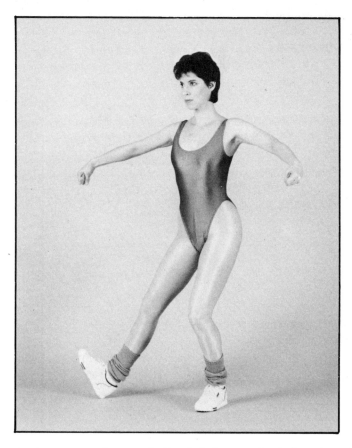

4. Repeat and stretch the left leg to the left side as the arms lift.

Continually changing legs, do 32 times.

Variation

You can move forward and backward as you do the half jack by slightly adjusting the placement of your feet. To walk forward, stretch the right leg to the side as above. Then cross the right foot, slightly turned

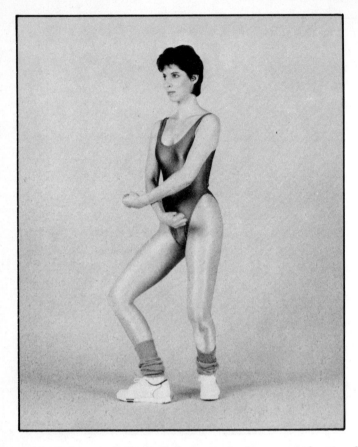

out, in front of the left foot and place weight on the foot. Continue by extending the left leg to the left side and crossing it in front of the right.

Walking backward is easy too! Simply cross the moving leg behind you, place weight on it and continue by extending the other leg to the side.

Walk forward for four steps and back for four steps.

Repeat four times.

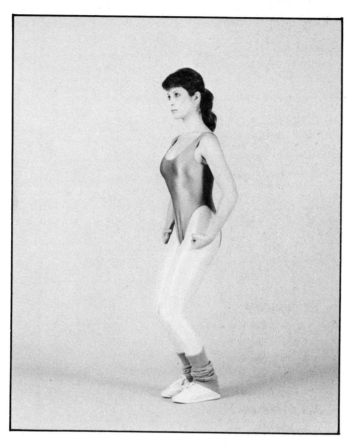

HEEL TOUCH/BICEPS BUILDER

1. Stand with legs together and knees slightly bent. Arms are down by sides with hands closed into fists.

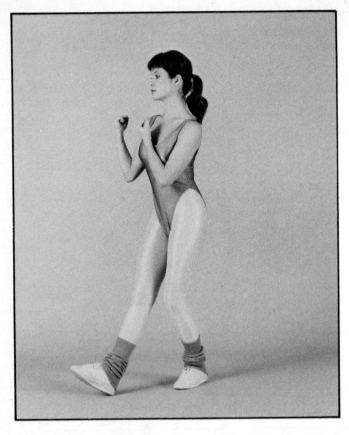

2. Extend the right leg forward and touch right heel
   to the floor with toes pointing up. At the same
   time, angle the arms to the right and bend the
   elbows to do a biceps curl. Bring the fists toward
   the shoulders in a controlled motion.
3. Lower the forearms as you return the right leg to
   the starting position.
4. Repeat by extending the left leg forward and
   angling the arms to the left.

Do 24 times, alternating legs.

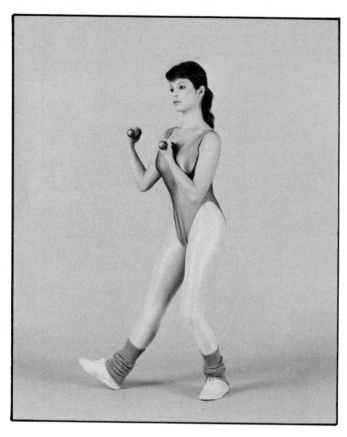

Variation

Extend the right leg to the side and touch heel to the floor. Alternate legs and repeat biceps curls.

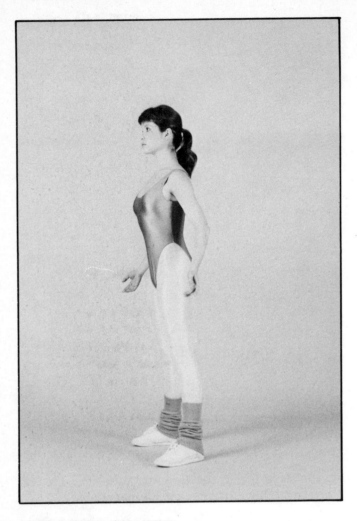

THE SPEED SKATER

1. Stand with feet shoulder-width apart, arms at
   sides.

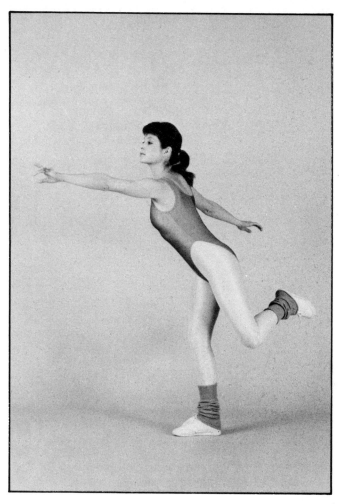

2. Place weight on the right foot and bend the right
   knee. At the same time, sweep the left foot off the
   floor as the left knee bends behind the body. The
   torso leans forward and the left arm lifts forward
   to shoulder height with a controlled swing as the
   right arm swings behind the body.

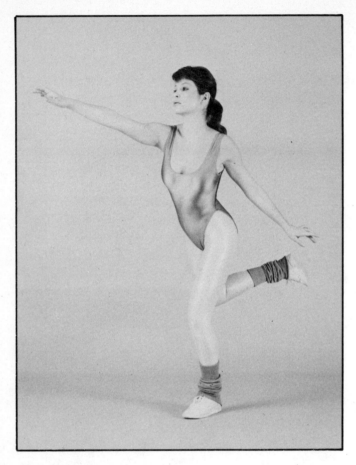

3. Change legs and arms and continue repeating the
   movement.

Repeat 32 times.

Variation

Change directions with the Speed Skater every eight
counts by making a quarter turn to the right and repeating the skating movement.

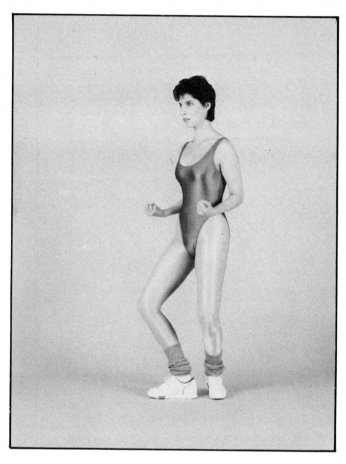

KARATE PUNCH

1. Place the right foot in front of the left foot with knees bent and the feet turned out. Bend both elbows into the waist and make fists.

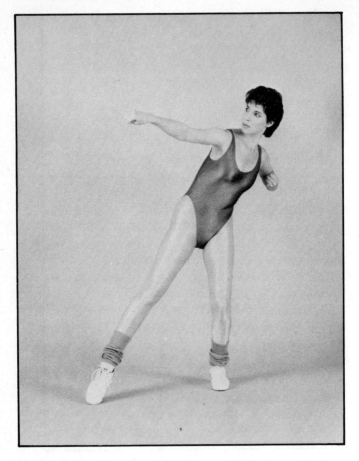

2. Raise the right heel and touch the toes of the right
   foot to the floor in front of the body as the torso
   and hips turn to face the left direction. At the
   same time, the right arm extends to the front and
   the fist pushes forward with a controlled punch.
   The left elbow bends and presses back.
3. Bring the feet together by bending the right knee
   and pulling the right heel toward the left toes.
   Bend both elbows into the waist.

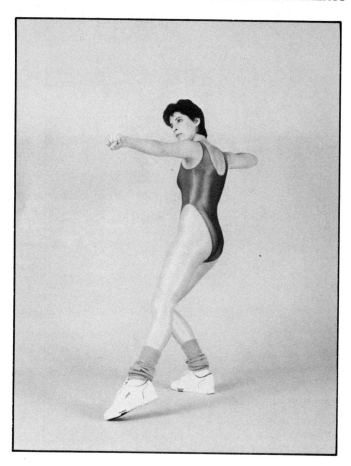

4. Repeat to the left side by extending the left leg in front of the body and turning the torso and hips to the right. The left arm pushes forward and the right elbow presses back.

Alternating sides, do 32.

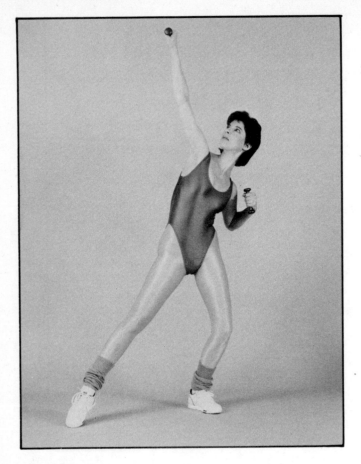

Variation

Punch the right arm to the ceiling when the right leg extends front. As the movement alternates sides, the left arm punches to the ceiling when the left leg extends front.

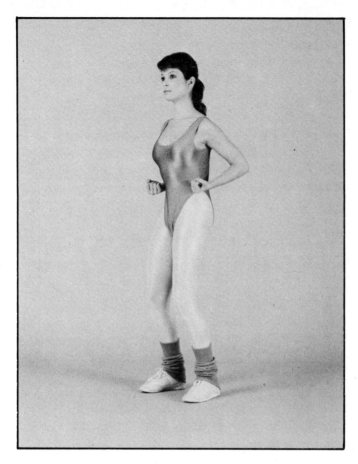

SIDE-TO-SIDE TOE TAP

1. Start with the feet hip-width apart and knees slightly bent. The arms are bent with the wrists at the waistline and the elbows behind the torso.
2. Keeping the knees bent, take a step to the right with the right foot.

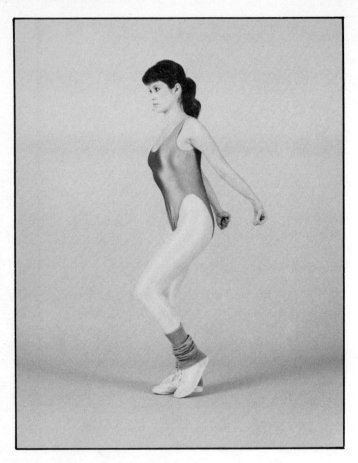

3. Tap the ball of the left foot next to the right. At the same time, extend the forearms behind the torso without moving the elbows. Do not lock or jam the elbows.
4. Step to the left and return the forearms to the starting position—elbows bent and wrists at the waist.
5. Tap the ball of the right foot next to the left foot and extend forearms behind torso.

Repeat 24 times.

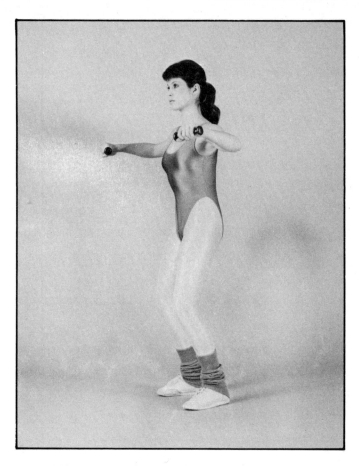

Variation

In the starting position, place the arms parallel to the floor with the elbows bent. Step to the right. As you tap the ball of the left foot, extend the arms forward and straighten the elbows. Repeat the same arm movement to the left.

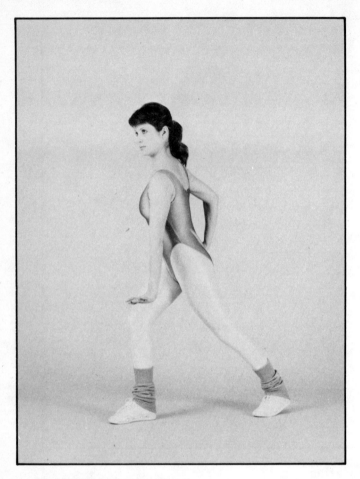

JAZZ PRESS-DOWN

1. Turning the body to the right, bend the right knee and extend left leg back to form a lunge position. At the same time, straighten the left arm and press the palm toward the floor. Bend the right elbow behind the torso.

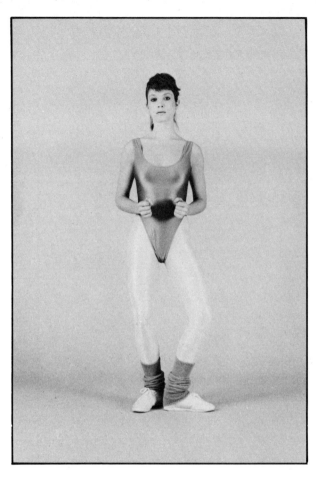

2. Slide the left foot in front of the right foot; both feet are turned out and knees bent. Bend the elbows and pull forearms into the waist.

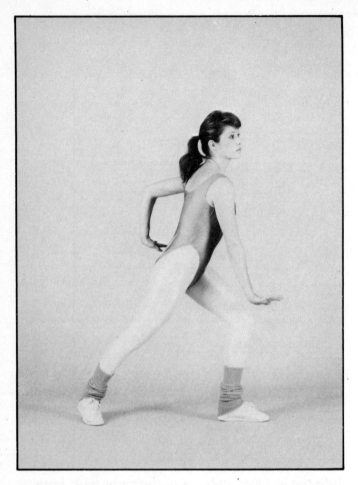

3. Turn to the left, bend the left knee and step the
   right foot out to the side to form the lunge
   position. Straighten the right arm and press the
   palm toward the floor as the left elbow bends
   behind the torso.

Changing from side to side, repeat 24 times.

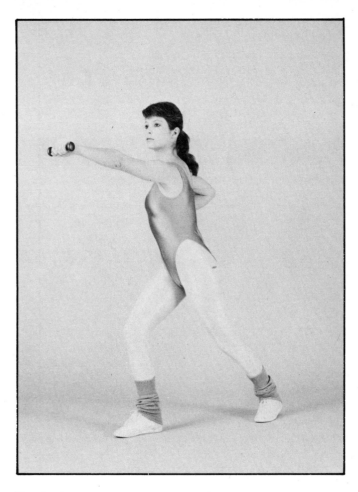

Variation

As you turn the body to the right, extend the left arm in front of the body. Repeat to the left side.

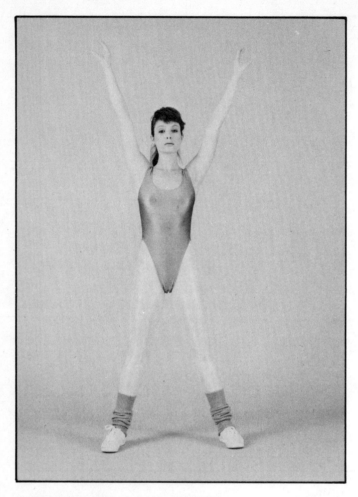

ELBOW-KNEE CONNECTION

1. Stand with feet shoulder-width apart, legs
   straight and knees relaxed. Arms are extended
   above the head in a V-shape.

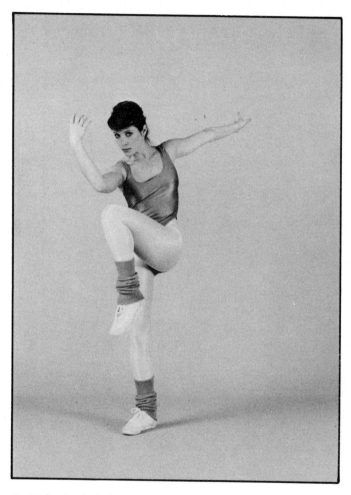

2. Lift the left knee toward the right bent elbow. (The elbow and knee do not have to touch.) Keep left arm straight and lower it to shoulder level.
3. Return to the starting position.
4. Repeat by lifting right knee to left elbow.

Alternating sides, do 24 total.

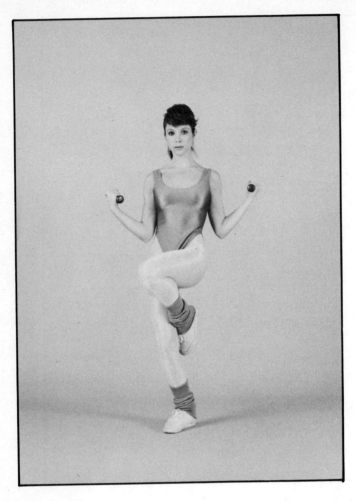

Variation

As each knee lifts, pull both elbows down (think of resisting against the air) toward the waist.

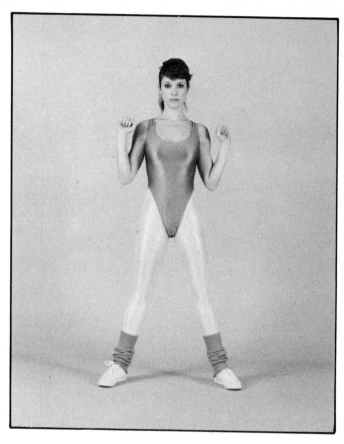

TOE TAPBACK

1. Starting with straight legs (knees are relaxed) and
   feet slightly wider than shoulder-width, bend
   arms and place hands in front of the shoulders.

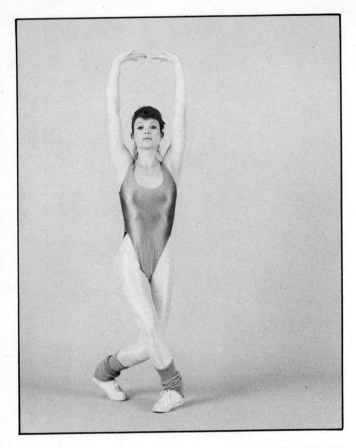

2. Bend the right knee and tap the ball of the left
   foot behind the right foot. At the same time,
   straighten the arms and push the palms toward
   the ceiling, fingers toward each other.
3. Bring the hands back to the shoulders as the legs
   return to the starting position.
4. Repeat to the left side. The accent of the
   movement is on the toe tap and the arms pushing
   up.

Alternating the legs, do 16 repetitions.

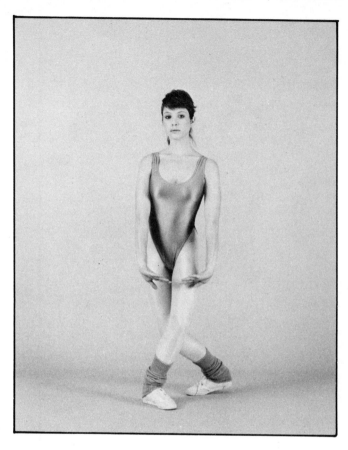

Variation

Each time the toe taps, push the hands down toward the floor (fingers toward each other) and straighten the arms.

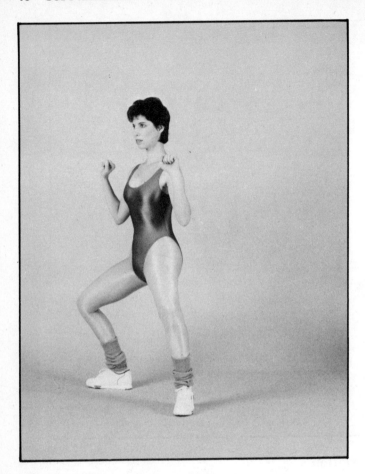

BEND STRETCH REACHER

1. Standing with feet about shoulder-width apart, bend the knees. Elbows are bent at waist with hands in front of shoulders.
2. Straighten both legs as you slide the left foot in to meet the right foot. At the same time, reach the

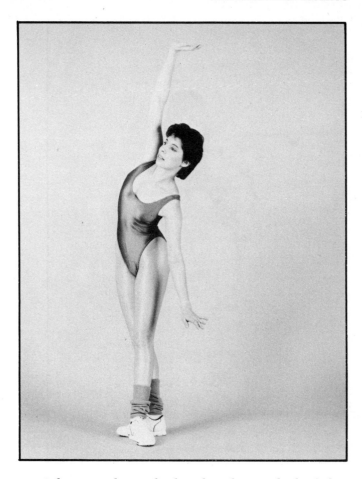

right arm above the head and stretch the left arm down.

3. Return to the starting position by stepping to the left side with the left foot, bending the knees and bringing the hands back to the shoulders with elbows bent.

4. Repeat the movement to the left side.

Continue alternating sides and do a total of 16.

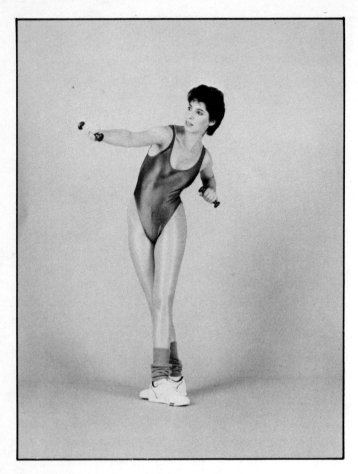

Variation

Instead of reaching the arm overhead, push the right arm straight ahead in front of the chest as the left elbow presses back.

7
THE ROUTINES

The following four routines incorporate the preceding twelve basic movements into a fifteen-minute soft aerobics workout. Each routine is slightly under four minutes. The workout is effective without weights for cardiovascular conditioning, but weights may be added to increase intensity for the well-conditioned exerciser.

To perform the workout with ease, take a few minutes to read through the entire pattern of gestures for each routine. Familiarize yourself with the movements and their variations. In some cases, leg movements are done without arm motions. This allows a smoother transition between steps and also gives the arm muscles a rest after a high number of repetitions. If a transition between two movements is difficult for you, stop for a moment to orient yourself to the next step. It can be helpful to practice a routine by first performing it slowly without music.

Once you're ready to start dancing, remember to monitor your heart rate between routines. If your pulse is higher than your specified target zone, decrease the intensity of your movements. Conversely, increase the intensity if you have not reached 60 percent of your maximum heart rate (220 minus your age). You can lower your heart rate by using less force and making your leg and arm movements smaller. The heart rate can be increased by making motions larger and applying greater force.

After completing the Low-Impact Workout, you may want to try developing your own soft aerobics routines. You can combine the twelve core movements in different patterns or create your own movements for new routines. Your inspiration for new steps may come from a snappy, upbeat piece of music that makes you want to move. Or, you might want to create new variations from the core movements by changing arm motions or foot patterns.

ROUTINE #1

Movement	Number of Repetitions
1. a. Pendulum Push—legs only	12
b. Pendulum Push—legs and arms	12
c. Pendulum Push Variation	12
2. a. Side-to-Side Toe Tap—legs only	12
b. Side-to-Side Toe Tap—legs and arms	24
3. a. Elbow-Knee Connection—legs only	12
b. Elbow-Knee Connection—legs and arms	12
4. Heel Touch/Biceps Builder	24
5. a. Half Jacks	24
b. Half Jacks Variation—walk forward four steps, walk backward four steps	4
6. a. Pendulum Push	12
b. Pendulum Push Variation—legs only	12
c. Repeat a.	12
d. Repeat b.	12
7. a. Side-to-Side Toe Tap—legs only	12
b. Side-to-Side Toe Tap—legs and arms	24

ROUTINE #2

Movement	Number of Repetitions
1. a. Bend Stretch Reacher—legs only	16
b. Bend Stretch Reacher—legs and arms	16
c. Repeat a.	8
d. Repeat b.	8
2. a. Chorus Line Special—legs only	16
b. Chorus Line Special—legs and arms	16
3. a. Karate Punch—legs only	8
b. Karate Punch—legs and arms	8
c. Karate Punch Variation	16
4. a. Half Jacks—legs only	8
b. Half Jacks—legs and arms	8
c. Half Jacks Variation—walk forward four steps, walk backward four steps	4
5. a. The Pull-Down Knee Lift—legs only	12
b. The Pull-Down Knee Lift—legs and arms	12
6. a. Chorus Line Special—legs only	16
b. Chorus Line Special Variation	16
7. a. Bend Stretch Reacher—legs only	16
b. Bend Stretch Reacher—legs and arms	16
8. a. Karate Punch—legs only	8
b. Karate Punch—legs and arms	8

ROUTINE #3

Movement	Number of Repetitions
1. a. Toe Tapback—legs only	16
b. Toe Tapback—legs and arms	16
c. Toe Tapback Variation	16
2. a. Speed Skater	8
b. Speed Skater Variation—four quarter turns, eight counts each direction	32
3. a. Pendulum Push—legs and arms	16
b. Pendulum Push Variation	16
4. a. Jazz Press-Down—legs only	8
b. Jazz Press-Down—legs and arms	16
c. Jazz Press-Down Variation	8
5. a. Bend Stretch Reacher—legs only	16
b. Bend Stretch Reacher Variation	16
6. a. Side-to-Side Toe Tap—legs only	8
b. Side-to-Side Toe Tap Variation	16
7. a. Toe Tapback—legs only	8
b. Toe Tapback—legs and arms	8
c. Toe Tapback Variation	8
d. Repeat a.	4
e. Repeat b.	4
f. Repeat c.	4
8. Speed Skater	16

ROUTINE #4

Movement	Number of Repetitions
1. a. Heel Touch/Biceps Builder—legs only	16
b. Heel Touch/Biceps Builder—legs and arms	16
c. Heel Touch/Biceps Builder Variation	16
2. a. Elbow-Knee Connection—legs only	8
b. Elbow-Knee Connection—legs and arms	16
3. a. Karate Punch	8
b. Karate Punch Variation	8
c. Repeat a.	8
d. Repeat b.	8
4. a. Pull-Down Knee Lift—legs only	8
b. Pull-Down Knee Lift—legs and arms	8
5. a. Bend Stretch Reacher—legs only	16
b. Bend Stretch Reacher Variation	16
6. a. Toe Tapback—legs only	16
b. Toe Tapback Variation	16
7. a. Heel Touch/Biceps Builder—legs only	8
b. Heel Touch/Biceps Builder Variation—legs only	8
c. Repeat a.—legs and arms	8
d. Repeat b.—legs and arms	8
8. Speed Skater Variation—four quarter turns, eight counts each direction	32
9. Half Jacks	24

8
THE COOL DOWN

No aerobic workout is complete without a cool down that gradually lowers the elevated heart rate and prevents muscles from stiffening. After you've performed the low-impact routines, it's crucial *not* to stop moving abruptly. You need to reduce your intensity level gradually to keep the blood pumping from the arms and legs back to the heart. When motion is suddenly stopped, blood can pool in the extremities resulting in lightheadedness, dizziness or fainting.

To decrease your intensity following the low-impact routines, repeat the Walk Around you used as a warm-up and select a slower-paced song to accompany your movement. The Walk Around should be done for three to five minutes during this recovery period. After completing the walk, check your pulse for a recovery heart rate. After five minutes of a cool down, your heart rate should be less than 60 percent of your maximum. If it is higher, continue walking slowly until it drops to the appropriate level. The recovery heart rate is an indicator of fitness. The sooner your heart returns to a resting level, the more conditioned you are.

Complete the cool down with a few more exercises to stretch muscles that were contracted during your soft aerobics routines. Don't overlook these final stretches, which are essential in preventing the muscles from becoming stiff and sore the day after a workout.

THE STRETCHES

These warm-up stretches are valuable to repeat during the cool down:

Spine Stretch
Shoulder Rotations
Deltoid Stretch
Triceps Stretch
Torso Stretch
Calf Stretch

In addition to the above exercises, include the following stretches:

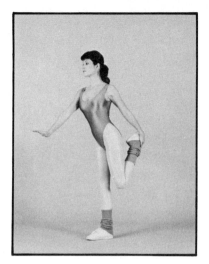 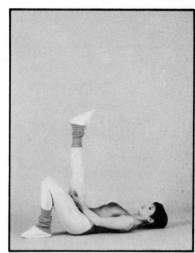

QUADRICEPS (FRONT OF THIGH) STRETCH

1. Standing on the right leg, bend left leg behind you and clasp instep with left hand. If necessary, hold on to a chair for balance. Keep the stomach pulled in and the pelvis vertical to prevent the back from arching.
2. Press the instep into the hand to increase the stretch in the front of the thigh. Hold for 15 seconds.
3. Change legs and repeat.

HAMSTRING STRETCH

1. Lying on the back, bend left knee and extend the right leg to the ceiling. Place hands on thigh and gently pull leg toward chest. Hold stretch for 20 seconds.
2. Repeat with left leg extended.

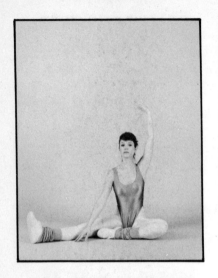 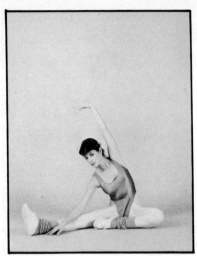

STRADDLE STRETCH

1. Sitting with the right leg extended to the side, bend the left leg and place the sole of the foot toward the right thigh. Stretch the left arm above the head and place the right arm on the inside of the right leg. Inhale.
2. Exhale and tilt the torso over the right leg. Hold stretch for 15 seconds.
3. Change legs and repeat to the left.

9
AEROBIC EXERCISE: WEIGHT CONTROL AND HEALTH

For many of us, the morning that we can't button a favorite skirt or expensive pair of trousers because our waistline has expanded is the morning we vow to lose weight. Sometimes we choose a diet so restricted in calories that it's difficult to follow, or we select an exercise program so rigorous and intense that it's hard to stick with the regimen. Misconceptions about weight control abound, and these notions about dieting and exercise for weight loss can lead to frustration and despair. Aerobic Exercise and Weight Control can help you develop a sensible and healthy approach to losing weight.

BODY FAT

Although most people develop weight-loss goals based on a number on the bathroom scale, an understanding of body composition can provide a truer assessment. Body composition refers to the amount of fat tissue in relation to lean body mass—the bones, muscles, organs and connective tissue. Body fat is necessary, but most of us have too much. While the scale gives a numerical figure for body weight, it cannot give the ratio of body fat to lean mass.

How can you measure body fat? There are a number of sophisticated techniques that can gauge body fat levels, but the skin caliper method may be most accessible. The caliper is an instrument that measures skin-fold thickness and the amount of fat immediately below the skin. Your physician may be able to do this measure for you. A more informal method is to grasp the flesh at the waistline or the back of the arm. If you can, as the saying goes, "pinch more than an inch," it's generally an indication that you are carrying too much fat.

Optimum fat level is based on the total of essential fat and stored fat. Essential fat is stored in the organs and various tissues and is required for normal functioning of the body. Men carry about 3 percent of their total body weight in essential fat. For women, essential fat includes an additional 9 percent of body weight in what is referred to as sex-specific or hormonally related fat.

Stored fat is the body fat that is found between the muscles and the skin. This fat acts as a concentrated store of energy to regulate body temperature and to protect the muscles, bones and organs from injury. Stored fat levels in men and women are similar, about 12 to 15 percent of total body weight.

Combining essential and stored fat, the desired fat level for men is 15 to 20 percent and for women 20 to 25 percent. When body fat exceeds these levels, it is evidence that there is too much stored fat. Obesity is considered a health risk factor when body fat levels are higher than 20 percent for men and 30 percent for women.

Fat accumulates when an energy imbalance exists—more calories are consumed than expended in activity. To maintain your weight, you must have a caloric intake equal to your caloric expenditure. Losing weight requires that more calories be expended than consumed.

DIET AND EXERCISE

Fact: Dieting alone is not the key to weight and fat control.

When your caloric intake is severely restricted, an interesting phenomenon occurs: the body thinks it is being starved. The results of this "starvation" are twofold. One, the body's metabolism actually decreases (it burns calories at a slower rate) to conserve the limited amount of fuel it is receiving. And two, when a diet is extremely low in calories, over time the body uses not only fat tissue to survive but lean body mass as well.

Fact: Short spurts of high-intensity exercise are ineffective fat burners.

Although it might seem that high-intensity activity would burn more fat, moderate activity is actually the more effective method for losing fat. Fat can only be used as a fuel source during aerobic activity. When the body works at very high intensity levels, aerobic metabolism (using oxygen for energy production) is replaced by anaerobic metabolism (energy production that can occur without oxygen). Exercise becomes anaerobic when you work above 85 percent of your maximum heart rate. Anaerobic metabolism does not use fat but rather carbohydrates and protein for fuel sources. When you exercise at an intensity of 60 to 75 percent, you are working hard enough to achieve cardiovascular benefits but also at a level that is low enough to use fat reserves for the major fuel source.

Losing fat and controlling your weight can best be achieved by combining a sound diet (no less than 1200 calories for women and 1600 calories for men) with lots of aerobic activity. Regular exercise will actually raise your metabolic rate because increased lean body mass burns calories at a higher rate than fat tissue. While exercising three times weekly is the minimum for cardiovascular conditioning, H D E (healthy doses of exercise!) is the prescription for losing weight. Five or six days per week at 60 to 75 percent intensity for 20 to 40 minutes per session will result in a significant loss of fat while preserving lean body mass. Remember to build the duration and frequency of your workouts gradually if you're a newcomer to exercise.

EXERCISE AND OSTEOPOROSIS

Not exercising is hazardous to your health!

This statement is a powerful warning to every woman concerned about developing osteoporosis, the crippling disease of the bones. One out of every four women over the age of 65 will develop osteoporosis, and, while the disease is not curable, it may be preventable. With foresight and information about exercise and nutrition, it is possible to keep your bones healthy and stay active throughout your life.

Osteoporosis means porous bones. As the disease develops, the bones become so thin and brittle that they break easily. Spine, wrist and hip fractures are the most common occurrences. Loss of calcium from the vertebral bones also causes the decrease in height experienced by some women as they age. Although there is a natural tendency for our bones to become weaker as we get older, osteoporosis exacerbates the process.

Over 15 million Americans have some degree of osteoporosis. It is a "silent" disease that progresses slowly, and it may be years or even decades before you know that you have it. Osteoporosis is eight times more common in women than in men, and it is most prevalent in Caucasian and Oriental women. You may be a likely candidate if you are small-boned, smoke, drink alcohol excessively, do not get adequate amounts of calcium in your diet and are sedentary.

As you age, the body takes calcium from the bones more rapidly than you can replace it. The process occurs even more quickly after menopause. Up to the age of 40, you can make the bones denser and stronger, but after 40, you can only slow down the rate of bone loss.

The critical factor in preventing osteoporosis is bone mass because stronger bones are less likely to break. Exercise thickens the bones by putting more calcium in them. People who are physically active throughout their lives have more bone mass than individuals with sedentary lifestyles. Inactivity and a lack of weight-bearing exercise contribute to bone loss while the effects of gravity and the muscle pull exerted on the bones during exercise create denser, stronger bones. This was documented in studies done during space travel with astronauts who showed a temporary loss of bone mass due to weightlessness.

Soft aerobics, along with other activities such as walking, social dancing and sports, do help create stronger bones because they are weight bearing. Additionally, the use of light weights for the upper body will help to thicken the arm bones. Although an activity such as swimming is beneficial to the cardiovascular system, the buoyance of the water supporting the body makes swimming ineffective in the prevention of osteoporosis.

To counteract osteoporosis, exercise and nutrition go hand in hand. Exercise can thicken and strengthen the bones only if you have enough calcium in your diet. Premenopausal women need 1000 milligrams of calcium daily; pregnant and nursing women require 1200 milligrams; and 1500 milligrams are recommended for postmenopausal females. The primary sources of calcium are milk and dairy products (one glass of milk provides approximately 300 milligrams). Calcium is also present in some leafy green vegetables and in canned salmon and sardines, if processed with their bones. Smaller amounts of calcium are available in other foods such as tofu, beans and oysters. If you do not get enough calcium through the foods you eat, you may need to add a vitamin supplement.

Osteoporosis does not need to affect the quality of your life in the later years. With regular exercise and sufficient calcium in your diet, you may have some control over the aging process.